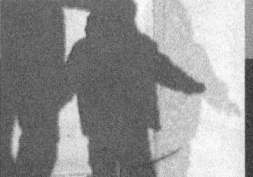

I0469485

Contents

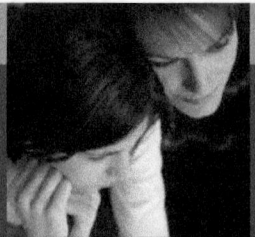

All parents can relate to the many changes their kids go through as they grow up. But sometimes it's hard to tell if a child is just going through a "phase," or perhaps showing signs of something more serious.

Recently, doctors have been diagnosing more children with bipolar disorder,[1] sometimes called manic-depressive illness. But what does this illness really mean for a child?

This booklet is a guide for parents who think their child may have symptoms of bipolar disorder, or parents whose child has been diagnosed with the illness.

This booklet discusses bipolar disorder in children and teens. For information on bipolar disorder in adults, see the National Institute of Mental Health (NIMH) booklet "Bipolar Disorder."

What is bipolar disorder?

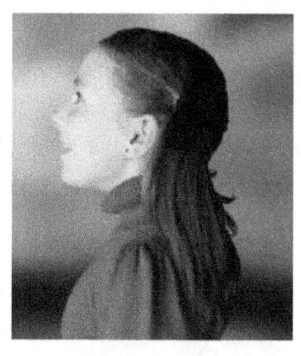

Bipolar disorder, also known as manic-depressive illness, is a brain disorder that causes unusual shifts in mood and energy. It can also make it hard for someone to carry out day-to-day tasks, such as going to school or hanging out with friends. Symptoms of bipolar disorder are severe. They are different from the normal ups and downs that everyone goes through from time to time. They can result in damaged relationships, poor school performance, and even suicide. But bipolar disorder can be treated, and people with this illness can lead full and productive lives.

Bipolar disorder often develops in a person's late teens or early adult years, but some people have their first symptoms during childhood. At least half of all cases start before age 25.[2]

What are common symptoms of bipolar disorder in children and teens?

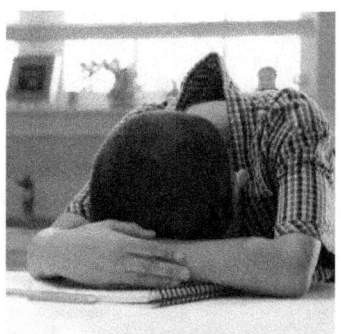

Youth with bipolar disorder experience unusually intense emotional states that occur in distinct periods called "mood episodes." An overly joyful or overexcited state is called a manic episode, and an extremely sad or hopeless state is called a depressive episode. Sometimes, a mood episode includes symptoms of both mania and depression. This is called a mixed state. People with bipolar disorder also may be explosive and irritable during a mood episode.

Extreme changes in energy, activity, sleep, and behavior go along with these changes in mood. Symptoms of bipolar disorder are described on the following page.

Symptoms of mania include:

Mood Changes

- Being in an overly silly or joyful mood that's unusual for your child. It is different from times when he or she might usually get silly and have fun.
- Having an extremely short temper. This is an irritable mood that is unusual.

Behavioral Changes

- Sleeping little but not feeling tired
- Talking a lot and having racing thoughts
- Having trouble concentrating, attention jumping from one thing to the next in an unusual way
- Talking and thinking about sex more often
- Behaving in risky ways more often, seeking pleasure a lot, and doing more activities than usual.

Symptoms of depression include:

Mood Changes

- Being in a sad mood that lasts a long time
- Losing interest in activities they once enjoyed
- Feeling worthless or guilty.

Behavioral Changes

- Complaining about pain more often, such as headaches, stomach aches, and muscle pains
- Eating a lot more or less and gaining or losing a lot of weight
- Sleeping or oversleeping when these were not problems before
- Losing energy
- Recurring thoughts of death or suicide.

It's normal for almost every child or teen to have some of these symptoms sometimes. These passing changes should not be confused with bipolar disorder.

Symptoms of bipolar disorder are not like the normal changes in mood and energy that everyone has now and then. Bipolar symptoms are more extreme and tend to last for most of the day, nearly every day, for at least one week. Also, depressive or manic episodes include moods very different from a child's normal mood, and the behaviors described in the chart above may start at the same time. Sometimes the symptoms of bipolar disorder are so severe that the child needs to be treated in a hospital.

In addition to mania and depression, bipolar disorder can cause a range of moods, as shown on the scale below. One side of the scale includes severe depression, moderate depression, and mild low mood. Moderate depression may cause less extreme symptoms, and mild low mood is called dysthymia when it is chronic or long-term. In the middle of the scale is normal or balanced mood.

	normal or balanced mood	
severe depression, moderate depression, and mild low mood		hypomania and severe mania

Sometimes, a child may have more energy and be more active than normal, but not show the severe signs of a full-blown manic episode. When this happens, it is called hypomania, and it generally lasts for at least four days in a row. Hypomania causes noticeable changes in behavior, but does not harm a child's ability to function in the way mania does.

What affects a child's risk of getting bipolar disorder?

Bipolar disorder tends to run in families. Children with a parent or sibling who has bipolar disorder are four to six times more likely to develop the illness, compared with children who do not have a family history of bipolar disorder.[3] However, most children with a family history of bipolar disorder will not develop the illness. Compared with children whose parents do not have bipolar disorder, 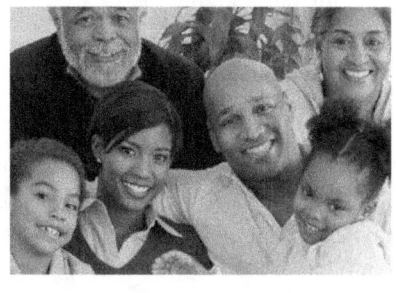 children whose parents have bipolar disorder may be more likely to have symptoms of anxiety disorders and attention deficit hyperactivity disorder (ADHD).[4]

Several studies show that youth with anxiety disorders are more likely to develop bipolar disorder than youth without anxiety disorders. However, anxiety disorders are very common in young people. Most children and teens with anxiety disorders do not develop bipolar disorder.[5, 6]

At this time, there is no way to prevent bipolar disorder. NIMH is currently studying how to limit or delay the first symptoms in children with a family history of the illness.

Also see the section in this booklet called "What illnesses often co-exist with bipolar disorder in children and teens?"

How does bipolar disorder affect children and teens differently than adults?

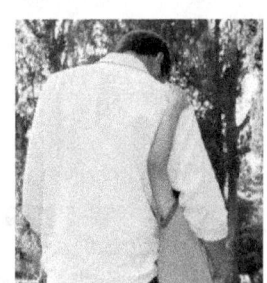

Bipolar disorder that starts during childhood or during the teen years is called early-onset bipolar disorder. Early-onset bipolar disorder seems to be more severe than the forms that first appear in older teens and adults.[7, 8] Youth with bipolar disorder are different from adults with bipolar disorder. Young people with the illness appear to have more frequent mood switches, are sick more often, and have more mixed episodes.[8]

Watch out for any sign of suicidal thinking or behaviors. Take these signs seriously. On average, people with early-onset bipolar disorder have greater risk for attempting suicide than those whose symptoms start in adulthood.[7, 9] One large study on bipolar disorder in children and teens found that more than one-third of study participants made at least one serious suicide attempt.[10] Some suicide attempts are carefully planned and others are not. Either way, it is important to understand that suicidal feelings and actions are symptoms of an illness that **must** be treated.

For more information on suicide, see the NIMH publication, *Suicide in the U.S.: Statistics and Prevention* on the NIMH Web site at http://www.nimh.nih.gov/health/publications/suicide-in-the-us-statistics-and-prevention.shtml.

How is bipolar disorder detected in children and teens?

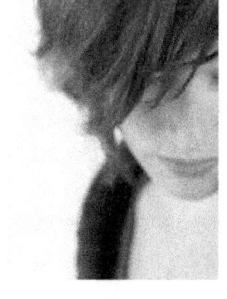

No blood tests or brain scans can diagnose bipolar disorder. However, a doctor may use tests like these to help rule out other possible causes for your child's symptoms. For example, the doctor may recommend testing for problems in learning, thinking, or speech and language.[11] A careful medical exam may also detect problems that commonly co-occur with bipolar disorder and need to be treated, such as substance abuse.

Doctors who have experience with diagnosing early-onset bipolar disorder, such as psychiatrists, psychologists, or other mental health specialists, will ask questions about changes in your child's mood. They will also ask about sleep patterns, activity or energy levels, and if your child has had any other mood or behavioral disorders. The doctor may also ask whether there is a family history of bipolar disorder or other psychiatric illnesses, such as depression or alcoholism.

Doctors usually diagnose mental disorders using guidelines from the *Diagnostic and Statistical Manual of Mental Disorders*, or DSM. According to the DSM, there are four basic types of bipolar disorder:

1. **Bipolar I Disorder** is mainly defined by manic or mixed episodes that last at least seven days, or by manic symptoms that are so severe that the person needs immediate hospital care. Usually, the person also has depressive episodes, typically lasting at least two weeks. The symptoms of mania or depression must be a major change from the person's normal behavior.

2. **Bipolar II Disorder** is defined by a pattern of depressive episodes shifting back and forth with hypomanic episodes, but no full-blown manic or mixed episodes.

3. **Bipolar Disorder Not Otherwise Specified (BP-NOS)** is diagnosed when a person has symptoms of the illness that do not meet diagnostic criteria for either bipolar I or II. The symptoms may not last long enough, or the person may have too few symptoms, to be diagnosed with bipolar I or II. However, the symptoms are clearly out of the person's normal range of behavior.

4. **Cyclothymic Disorder, or Cyclothymia**, is a mild form of bipolar disorder. People who have cyclothymia have episodes of hypomania that shift back and forth with mild depression for at least two years (one year for children and adolescents). However, the symptoms do not meet the diagnostic requirements for any other type of bipolar disorder.

When children have manic symptoms that last for less than four days, experts recommend that they be diagnosed with BP-NOS. Some scientific evidence indicates that about one-third of these young people will develop longer episodes within a few years. If so, they meet the criteria for bipolar I or II.[12]

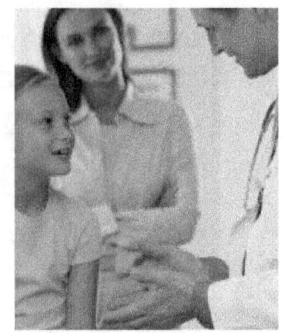

Also, researchers are working on whether certain symptoms mean a child should be diagnosed with bipolar disorder. For example, scientists are studying children with very severe, chronic irritability and symptoms of ADHD, but no clear episodes of mania. Some experts think these children should be diagnosed with mania. At the same time, there is scientific evidence that suggests these irritable children are different from children with bipolar disorder in the following key areas: the outcome of their illness, family history, and brain function.[13-16]

When you talk to your child's doctor or a mental health specialist, be sure to ask questions. Getting answers helps you understand the terms they use to describe your child's symptoms.

What illnesses often co-exist with bipolar disorder in children and teens?

Several illnesses may develop in people with bipolar disorder.

Alcoholism. Adults with bipolar disorder are at very high risk of developing a substance abuse problem. Young people with bipolar disorder may have the same risk.

ADHD. Many children with bipolar disorder have a history of ADHD.[17] One study showed that ADHD is more common in people whose bipolar disorder started during childhood, compared with people whose bipolar disorder started later in life.[7] Children who have co-occurring ADHD and bipolar disorder may have difficulty concentrating and controlling their activity. This may happen even when they are not manic or depressed.

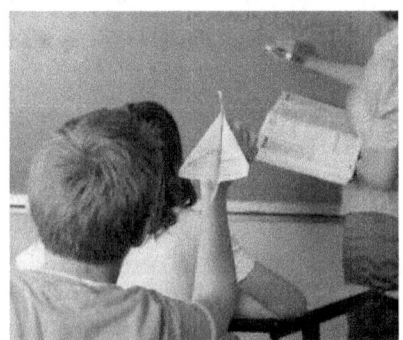

Anxiety Disorders. Anxiety disorders, such as separation anxiety and generalized anxiety disorder, also commonly co-occur with bipolar disorder. This may happen in both children and adults. Children who have both types of disorders tend to develop bipolar disorder at a younger age and have more hospital stays related to mental illness.[18]

Other Mental Disorders. Some mental disorders cause symptoms similar to bipolar disorder. Two examples are major depression (sometimes called unipolar depression) and ADHD. If you look at symptoms only, there is no way to tell the difference between major depression and a depressive episode in bipolar disorder. For this reason, be sure to tell a diagnosing doctor of any past manic symptoms or episodes your child may have had. In contrast, ADHD does not have episodes. ADHD symptoms may resemble mania in some ways, but they tend to be more constant than in a manic episode of bipolar disorder.

What treatments are available for children and teens with bipolar disorder?

To date, there is no cure for bipolar disorder. However, treatment with medications, psychotherapy (talk therapy), or both may help people get better.

It's important for you to know that children sometimes respond differently to psychiatric medications than adults do.

To treat children and teens with bipolar disorder, doctors often rely on information about treating adults. This is because there haven't been many studies on treating young people with the illness, although several have been started recently.

One large study with adults funded by NIMH is the Systematic Treatment Enhancement Program for Bipolar Disorder (STEP-BD—more information at http://www.nimh.nih.gov/health/trials/practical/step-bd/index.shtml). This study found that treating adults with medications and intensive psychotherapy for about nine months helped them get better. These adults got better faster and stayed well longer than adults treated with less intensive psychotherapy for six weeks.[19] Combining medication treatment and psychotherapies may help young people with early-onset bipolar disorder as well.[11] However, it's important for you to know that children sometimes respond differently to psychiatric medications than adults do.

Medications

Before starting medication, the doctor will want to determine your child's physical and mental health. This is called a "baseline" assessment. Your child will need regular follow-up visits to monitor treatment progress and side effects. Most children with bipolar disorder will also need long-term or even lifelong medication treatment. This is often the best way to manage symptoms and prevent relapse, or a return of symptoms.[11]

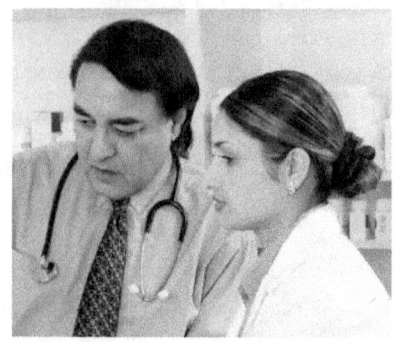

It's better to limit the number and dose of medications. A good way to remember this is "start low, go slow." Talk to the psychiatrist about using the smallest amount of medication that helps relieve your child's symptoms. To judge a medication's effectiveness, your child may need to take a medication for several weeks or months. The doctor needs this time to decide whether to switch to a different medication. Because children's symptoms are complex, it's not unusual for them to need more than one type of medication.[20]

Keep a daily log of your child's most troublesome symptoms. Doing so can make it easier for you, your child, and the doctor to decide whether a medication is helpful. Also, be sure to tell the psychiatrist about all other prescription drugs, over-the-counter medications, or natural supplements your child is taking. Taking certain medications and supplements together may cause unwanted or dangerous effects.

Some of the types of medications generally used to treat bipolar disorder are listed below. Information on medications can change. For the most up to date information on use and side effects contact the U.S. Food and Drug Administration (FDA) at http://www.fda.gov. You can also find more information in the NIMH Medications booklet at http://www.nimh.nih.gov/health/publications/medications/complete-publication.shtml.

To date, **lithium** (sometimes known as Eskalith), **risperidone** (Risperdal), and **aripiprazole** (Abilify) are the only medications approved by the U.S. Food and Drug Administration (FDA) to treat bipolar disorder in young people.

Lithium is a type of medication called a mood stabilizer. It can help treat and prevent manic symptoms[11] in children ages 12 and older.[21] In addition, there is some evidence that lithium might act as an antidepressant and help prevent suicidal behavior.[22] However, FDA's approval of lithium was based on treatment studies in adults. In fact, some experts say the FDA might not approve giving lithium to bipolar youth if the agency were to review this treatment today.

Risperidone and aripiprazole are a type of medication called an atypical, or second-generation, antipsychotic. These medications are called "atypical" to set them apart from earlier types of medications, called conventional or first generation antipsychotics. Short-term treatment with risperidone can help reduce symptoms of mania or mixed mania in children ages 10 and up. Aripiprazole is approved to treat these symptoms in children 10–17 years old who have bipolar I.[21]

Lithium Poisoning

Children may be showing early signs of lithium poisoning if they develop the following:

- Diarrhea

- Drowsiness

- Muscle weakness

- Lack of coordination

- Vomiting.

Take your child to the emergency room if he or she is taking lithium and has these symptoms. You should know that the risk of lithium poisoning goes up when a child becomes dehydrated. Make sure your child has enough to drink when he or she has a fever or sweats, such as when playing sports in the hot summer.

Your child's psychiatrist may recommend other types of medication, which are listed below. Studies in adults with bipolar disorder show these medications may be helpful. However, these medications have not been approved by the FDA to treat bipolar disorder in children.

Anticonvulsant medications are commonly prescribed to treat seizures, but these medications can help stabilize moods too. They may be very helpful for difficult-to-treat bipolar episodes. For some children, anticonvulsants may work better than lithium. Not every child can take lithium. Examples of anticonvulsant medications include:

- Valproic acid or divalproex sodium (Depakote)
- Lamotrigine (Lamictal).

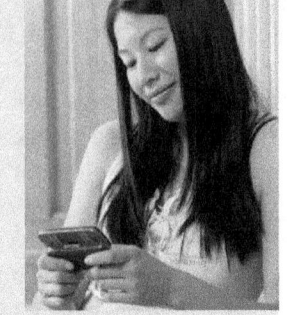
Valproic acid, lamotrigine, and other anticonvulsant medications have an FDA warning. The warning states that their use may increase the risk of suicidal thoughts and behaviors. People taking anticonvulsant medications for bipolar or other illnesses should be closely monitored for new or worsening symptoms of depression, suicidal thoughts or behavior, or any unusual changes in mood or behavior. People taking these medications should not make any changes without talking to their health care professional.

Atypical antipsychotic medications are sometimes used to treat symptoms of bipolar disorder in children. These medications are called "atypical" to set them apart from earlier types of medications, called conventional or first-generation antipsychotics. In addition to risperidone and aripiprazole, atypical antipsychotic medications include:

- Olanzapine (Zyprexa)
- Quetiapine (Seroquel)
- Ziprasidone (Geodon).

Antidepressant medications are sometimes used to treat symptoms of depression in bipolar disorder. Doctors who prescribe antidepressants for bipolar disorder usually prescribe a mood stabilizer or anticonvulsant medication at the same time. If your child takes only an antidepressant, he or she may be at risk of switching to mania or hypomania. He or she may also be at risk of developing rapid cycling symptoms.[26] Rapid cycling is when someone has four or more episodes of major depression, mania, hypomania, or mixed symptoms within a year.[27]

Some antidepressants that may be prescribed to treat symptoms of bipolar depression are:

- Fluoxetine (Prozac)
- Paroxetine (Paxil)
- Sertraline (Zoloft).

However, results on effectiveness of antidepressants for treating bipolar depression are mixed. The STEP-BD study showed that, in adults, adding an antidepressant to a mood stabilizer is no more effective in treating depression than using a mood stabilizer alone.[28]

FDA Warning on Antidepressants

Antidepressants are safe and popular, but some studies have suggested that they may have unintentional effects on some people, especially in adolescents and young adults. The FDA warning says that patients of all ages taking antidepressants should be watched closely, especially during the first few weeks of treatment. Possible side effects to look for are depression that gets worse, suicidal thinking or behavior, or any unusual changes in behavior such as trouble sleeping, agitation, or withdrawal from normal social situations. Families and caregivers should report any changes to the doctor. The latest information from the FDA can be found at http://www.fda.gov.

Some medications are better at treating one type of bipolar symptom than another. For example, lamotrigine (Lamictal) seems to be helpful in controlling depressive symptoms of bipolar disorder.[11]

What are the side effects of these medications?

Before your child starts taking a new medication, talk with the doctor or pharmacist about possible risks and benefits of taking that medication.

The doctor or pharmacist can also answer questions about side effects. Over the last decade, treatments have improved, and some medications now have fewer or more tolerable side effects than past treatments. However, everyone responds differently to medications, and in some cases, side effects may not appear until a person has taken a medication for some time.

If your child develops any severe side effects from a medication, talk to the doctor who prescribed it as soon as possible. The doctor may change the dose or prescribe a different medication. Children and teens being treated for bipolar disorder should not stop taking a medication without talking to a doctor first. Suddenly stopping a medication may lead to "rebound," or worsening of bipolar disorder symptoms or other uncomfortable or potentially dangerous withdrawal effects.

The following sections describe some common side effects of the different types of medications used to treat bipolar disorder.

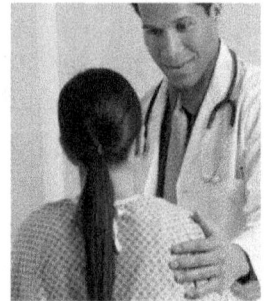

1. Mood Stabilizers

In some cases, lithium can cause side effects such as:

- Restlessness
- Frequent urination
- Dry mouth
- Bloating or indigestion
- Acne
- Joint or muscle pain
- Brittle nails or hair.[29]

Lithium may cause other side effects not listed here. Tell the doctor about bothersome or unusual side effects as soon as possible.

If your child is being treated with lithium, it is important for him or her to see the treating doctor regularly. The doctor needs to check the levels of lithium in the child's blood, as well as kidney function and thyroid function.

Each mood stabilizing medication is different and can cause different types of side effects. Some common side effects of lamotrigine and valproic acid include:

- Drowsiness
- Dizziness
- Headache
- Diarrhea
- Constipation
- Heartburn
- Mood swings
- Stuffed or runny nose, or other cold-like symptoms.[30, 31]

These medications may also be linked with rare but serious side effects. Talk with the treating doctor or a pharmacist to make sure you understand signs of serious side effects for the specific medications your child is taking.

2. Atypical Antipsychotics

Some people have side effects when they start taking atypical antipsychotics. Most side effects go away after a few days and often can be managed successfully. People who are taking antipsychotics should not drive until they adjust to their new medication. Side effects of many antipsychotics include:

- Drowsiness
- Dizziness when changing positions
- Blurred vision
- Rapid heartbeat
- Sensitivity to the sun
- Skin rashes
- Menstrual problems for girls
- Weight gain.

Atypical antipsychotic medications can cause major weight gain and changes in metabolism. This may increase a person's risk of getting diabetes and high cholesterol.[32] While taking an atypical antipsychotic medication, your child's weight, glucose levels, and lipid levels should be monitored regularly by a doctor.

In rare cases, long-term use of atypical antipsychotic drugs may lead to a condition called tardive dyskinesia (TD). The condition causes muscle movements that commonly occur around the mouth. A person with TD cannot control these movements. TD can range from mild to severe, and it cannot always be cured. Sometimes people with TD recover partially or fully after they stop taking the drug.

3. Antidepressants

The antidepressants most commonly prescribed for treating symptoms of bipolar disorder can also cause mild side effects that usually do not last long. These can include:

- Headache, which usually goes away within a few days.
- Nausea (feeling sick to your stomach), which usually goes away within a few days.

- Sleep problems, such as sleeplessness or drowsiness. This may occur during the first few weeks but then goes away. To help lessen these effects, sometimes the medication dose can be reduced, or the time of day it is taken can be changed.
- Agitation (feeling jittery).
- Sexual problems, which can affect both men and women. These include reduced sex drive and problems having and enjoying sex.

Some antidepressants are more likely to cause certain side effects than other antidepressants. Your doctor or pharmacist can answer questions about these medications. Any unusual reactions or side effects should be reported to a doctor immediately.

For the most up-to-date information on medications for treating bipolar disorder and their side effects, please see the online NIMH Medications booklet at http://www.nimh.nih.gov/health/publications/medications/complete-publication.shtml.

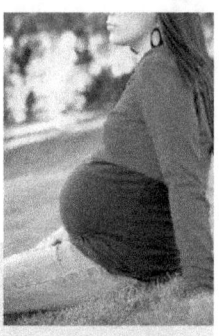

Sexual Activity, Pregnancy, and Teens with Bipolar Disorder

Many teens make risky choices about sex. The U.S. Centers for Disease Control and Prevention (CDC) recently reported that 26 percent of teenage girls in the United States have at least one of the four most common sexually transmitted diseases.[33] This suggests that many teens are having unprotected sex or taking part in other risky behaviors.

Bipolar disorder is also linked with impulsive and risky choices. Teenage girls with bipolar disorder who are pregnant or may become pregnant face special challenges because medications for the illness may have harmful effects on a developing fetus or nursing infant.[34] Specifically, lithium and valproic acid should not be used during pregnancy. Also, some medications may reduce the effectiveness of birth control pills.[35] For more information on managing bipolar disorder during and after pregnancy, see the NIMH booklet *Bipolar Disorder*.

Psychotherapy

In addition to medication, psychotherapy ("talk" therapy) can be an effective treatment for bipolar disorder. Studies in adults show that it can provide support, education, and guidance to people with bipolar disorder and their families. Psychotherapy may also help children keep taking their medications to stay healthy and prevent relapse.

> **Children and teens may also benefit from therapies that address problems at school, work, or in the community.**

Some psychotherapy treatments used for bipolar disorder include:

1. **Cognitive behavioral therapy** helps young people with bipolar disorder learn to change harmful or negative thought patterns and behaviors.
2. **Family-focused therapy** includes a child's family members. It helps enhance family coping strategies, such as recognizing new episodes early and helping their child. This therapy also improves communication and problem-solving.
3. **Interpersonal and social rhythm therapy** helps children and teens with bipolar disorder improve their relationships with others and manage their daily routines. Regular daily routines and sleep schedules may help protect against manic episodes.
4. **Psychoeducation** teaches young people with bipolar disorder about the illness and its treatment. This treatment helps people recognize signs of relapse so they can seek treatment early, before a full-blown episode occurs. Psychoeducation also may be helpful for family members and caregivers.

Other types of therapies may be tried as well, or used along with those mentioned above. The number, frequency, and type of psychotherapy sessions should be based on your child's treatment needs.

A licensed psychologist, social worker, or counselor typically provides these therapies. This professional often works with your child's psychiatrist to monitor care. Some may also be licensed to prescribe medications; check the laws in your state. For more information, see the Substance Abuse and Mental Health Services Administration Web page on choosing a mental health therapist at http://mentalhealth.samhsa.gov/publications/allpubs/KEN98-0046/default.asp.

In addition to getting therapy to reduce symptoms of bipolar disorder, children and teens may also benefit from therapies that address problems at school, work, or in the community. Such therapies may target communication skills, problem-solving skills, or skills for school or work. Other programs, such as those provided by social welfare programs or support and advocacy groups, can help as well.[11]

Some children with bipolar disorder may also have learning disorders or language problems.[36] Your child's school may need to make accommodations that reduce the stresses of a school day and provide proper support or interventions.

What can children and teens with bipolar disorder expect from treatment?

There is no cure for bipolar disorder, but it can be treated effectively over the long term. Doctors and families of children with bipolar disorder should keep track of symptoms and treatment effects to decide whether changes to the treatment plan are needed.

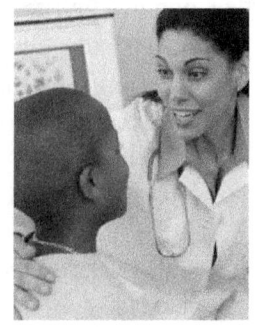

Sometimes a child may switch from one type of bipolar disorder to another. This calls for a change in treatment. In the largest study to date on childhood bipolar disorder, the NIMH-funded Course and Outcome of Bipolar Illness in Youth (COBY) study, researchers found that roughly one out of three children with BP-NOS later switched to bipolar I or II (see definitions on page 5). Also, roughly one out of five children who started out with a diagnosis of bipolar II switched to bipolar I.[8] Because different medications may be more helpful for one type of symptom than another (manic or depressive), your child may need to change medications or try different treatments if his or her symptoms change.

The COBY study also showed that treatment helped around 70 percent of children with bipolar disorder recover from their most recent episode (either manic or depressive). In this study, recovery meant having two or fewer symptoms for at least eight weeks in a row. On average, it took a little over a year and a half to recover. However, within the next year or so, symptoms returned in half of the children who recovered. Children with bipolar I or II tended to recover faster than those with BP-NOS, but their symptoms returned more frequently as well.

If your child has other psychiatric illnesses, such as an anxiety disorder, eating disorder, or substance abuse disorder, he or she may be more likely to experience a relapse — especially depressive symptoms.[37] Scientists are unsure how these co-existing illnesses increase the chance of relapse.

Working closely with your child's doctor and therapist and talking openly about treatment choices can make treatment more effective. You may need to talk about changing the treatment plan occasionally to help your child manage the illness most effectively.

For more information on psychotherapy, visit the NIMH Web site at http://www.nimh.nih.gov/health/topics/treatment/index.shtml.

Also, you may wish to keep a chart of your child's daily mood symptoms, treatments, sleep patterns, and life events, which can help you and your child better understand the illness. Sometimes this is called a mood chart or a daily life chart. It can help the doctor track and treat the illness more effectively. Examples of mood charts can be found on the Internet.

Where can families of children with bipolar disorder get help?

As with other serious illnesses, taking care of a child with bipolar disorder is incredibly hard on the parents, family, and other caregivers. Caregivers often must tend to the medical needs of their child while dealing with how it affects their own health. The stress that caregivers are under may lead to missed work or lost free time. It can strain relationships with people who do not understand the situation and lead to physical and mental exhaustion.

Stress from caregiving can make it hard to cope with your child's bipolar symptoms. One study shows that if a caregiver is under a lot of stress, his or her loved one has more trouble sticking to the treatment plan, which increases the chance for a major bipolar episode.[38] It is important to take care of your own physical and mental health. You may also find it helpful to join a local support group. If your child's illness prevents you from attending a local support group, try an online support group.

Where can I go for help?

If you are unsure where to go for help, ask your family doctor. Others who can help are listed below.

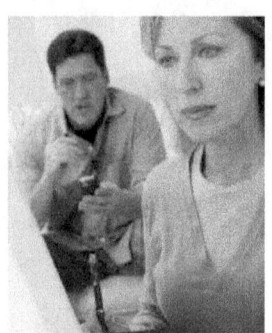

- Mental health specialists, such as psychiatrists, psychologists, social workers, or mental health counselors
- Health maintenance organizations
- Community mental health centers
- Hospital psychiatry departments and outpatient clinics
- Mental health programs at universities or medical schools
- State hospital outpatient clinics
- Family services, social agencies, or clergy
- Peer support groups
- Private clinics and facilities
- Employee assistance programs
- Local medical and/or psychiatric societies.

You can also check the phone book under "mental health," "health," "social services," "hotlines," or "physicians" for phone numbers and addresses. An emergency room doctor can also provide temporary help and can tell you where and how to get further help.

What if my child is in crisis?

If you think your child is in crisis:

- Call your doctor
- Call 911 or go to a hospital emergency room to get immediate help or ask a friend or family member to help you do these things
- Call the toll-free, 24-hour hotline of the National Suicide Prevention Lifeline at 1–800–273–TALK (1–800–273–8255); TTY: 1–800–799–4TTY (4889) to talk to a trained counselor
- Make sure your child is not left alone.

Citations

1. Moreno C, Laje G, Blanco C, Jiang H, Schmidt AB, Olfson M. National Trends in the Outpatient Treatment of Bipolar Disorder in Youth. *Arch Gen Psychiatry*. 2007 Sep;64(9):1032-1039.

2. Kessler RC, Berglund P, Demler O, Jin R, Merikangas KR, Walters EE. Lifetime prevalence and age-of-onset distributions of DSM-IV disorders in the National Comorbidity Survey Replication. *Arch Gen Psychiatry*. 2005 Jun;62(6):593-602.

3. Nurnberger JI, Jr., Foroud T. Genetics of bipolar affective disorder. *Curr Psychiatry Rep*. 2000 Apr;2(2):147-157.

4. Chang K, Steiner H, Ketter T. Studies of offspring of parents with bipolar disorder. *Am J Med Genet C Semin Med Genet*. 2003 Nov 15;123(1):26-35.

5. Johnson JG, Cohen P, Brook JS. Associations between bipolar disorder and other psychiatric disorders during adolescence and early adulthood: a community-based longitudinal investigation. *Am J Psychiatry*. 2000 Oct;157(10):1679-1681.

6. Bruckl TM, Wittchen HU, Hofler M, Pfister H, Schneider S, Lieb R. Childhood separation anxiety and the risk of subsequent psychopathology: Results from a community study. *Psychother Psychosom*. 2007 76(1):47-56.

7. Perlis RH, Miyahara S, Marangell LB, Wisniewski SR, Ostacher M, DelBello MP, Bowden CL, Sachs GS, Nierenberg AA. Long-term implications of early onset in bipolar disorder: data from the first 1000 participants in the systematic treatment enhancement program for bipolar disorder (STEP-BD). *Biol Psychiatry*. 2004 May 1;55(9):875-881.

8. Birmaher B, Axelson D, Strober M, Gill MK, Valeri S, Chiappetta L, Ryan N, Leonard H, Hunt J, Iyengar S, Keller M. Clinical course of children and adolescents with bipolar spectrum disorders. *Arch Gen Psychiatry*. 2006 Feb;63(2):175-183.

9. Bellivier F, Golmard JL, Henry C, Leboyer M, Schurhoff F. Admixture analysis of age at onset in bipolar I affective disorder. *Arch Gen Psychiatry*. 2001 May;58(5):510-512.

10. Goldstein TR, Birmaher B, Axelson D, Ryan ND, Strober MA, Gill MK, Valeri S, Chiappetta L, Leonard H, Hunt J, Bridge JA, Brent DA, Keller M. History of suicide attempts in pediatric bipolar disorder: factors associated with increased risk. *Bipolar Disord*. 2005 Dec;7(6):525-535.

11. McClellan J, Kowatch R, Findling RL. Practice parameter for the assessment and treatment of children and adolescents with bipolar disorder. *J Am Acad Child Adolesc Psychiatry*. 2007 Jan;46(1):107-125.

12. Axelson D, Birmaher B, Strober M, Gill MK, Valeri S, Chiappetta L, Ryan N, Leonard H, Hunt J, Iyengar S, Bridge J, Keller M. Phenomenology of children and adolescents with bipolar spectrum disorders. *Arch Gen Psychiatry*. 2006 Oct;63(10):1139-1148.

13. Tillman R, Geller B. Definitions of rapid, ultrarapid, and ultradian cycling and of episode duration in pediatric and adult bipolar disorders: a proposal to distinguish episodes from cycles. *J Child Adolesc Psychopharmacol*. 2003 Fall;13(3):267-271.

14. Brotman MA, Kassem L, Reising MM, Guyer AE, Dickstein DP, Rich BA, Towbin KE, Pine DS, McMahon FJ, Leibenluft E. Parental diagnoses in youth with narrow phenotype bipolar disorder or severe mood dysregulation. *Am J Psychiatry*. 2007 Aug;164(8):1238-1241.

15. Brotman MA, Schmajuk M, Rich BA, Dickstein DP, Guyer AE, Costello EJ, Egger HL, Angold A, Pine DS, Leibenluft E. Prevalence, clinical correlates, and longitudinal course of severe mood dysregulation in children. *Biol Psychiatry*. 2006 Nov 1;60(9):991-997.

16. Rich BA, Schmajuk M, Perez-Edgar KE, Fox NA, Pine DS, Leibenluft E. Different psychophysiological and behavioral responses elicited by frustration in pediatric bipolar disorder and severe mood dysregulation. *Am J Psychiatry*. 2007 Feb;164(2):309-317.

17. Tillman R, Geller B, Bolhofner K, Craney JL, Williams M, Zimerman B. Ages of onset and rates of syndromal and subsyndromal comorbid DSM-IV diagnoses in a prepubertal and early adolescent bipolar disorder phenotype. *J Am Acad Child Adolesc Psychiatry*. 2003 Dec;42(12):1486-1493.

18. Dickstein DP, Rich BA, Binstock AB, Pradella AG, Towbin KE, Pine DS, Leibenluft E. Comorbid anxiety in phenotypes of pediatric bipolar disorder. *J Child Adolesc Psychopharmacol*. 2005 Aug;15(4):534-548.

19. Miklowitz DJ, Otto MW, Frank E, Reilly-Harrington NA, Wisniewski SR, Kogan JN, Nierenberg AA, Calabrese JR, Marangell LB, Gyulai L, Araga M, Gonzalez JM, Shirley ER, Thase ME, Sachs GS. Psychosocial treatments for bipolar depression: a 1-year randomized trial from the Systematic Treatment Enhancement Program (STEP). *Arch Gen Psychiatry*. 2007 Apr;64(4):419-426.

20. Bhangoo RK, Lowe CH, Myers FS, Treland J, Curran J, Towbin KE, Leibenluft E. Medication use in children and adolescents treated in the community for bipolar disorder. *J Child Adolesc Psychopharmacol*. 2003 Winter;13(4):515-522.

21. U.S. Food and Drug Administration. Pediatric Exclusivity Labeling Changes http://www.fda.gov/cder/pediatric/labelchange.htm. Accessed on August 19, 2008.

22. Freeman MP, Freeman SA. Lithium: clinical considerations in internal medicine. *Am J Med*. 2006 Jun;119(6):478-481.

23. Vainionpaa LK, Rattya J, Knip M, Tapanainen JS, Pakarinen AJ, Lanning P, Tekay A, Myllyla VV, Isojarvi JI. Valproate-induced hyperandrogenism during pubertal maturation in girls with epilepsy. *Ann Neurol*. 1999 Apr;45(4):444-450.

24. Joffe H, Cohen LS, Suppes T, McLaughlin WL, Lavori P, Adams JM, Hwang CH, Hall JE, Sachs GS. Valproate is associated with new-onset oligoamenorrhea with hyperandrogenism in women with bipolar disorder. *Biol Psychiatry*. 2006 Jun 1;59(11):1078-1086.

25. Joffe H, Cohen LS, Suppes T, Hwang CH, Molay F, Adams JM, Sachs GS, Hall JE. Longitudinal follow-up of reproductive and metabolic features of valproate-associated polycystic ovarian syndrome features: A preliminary report. *Biol Psychiatry*. 2006 Dec 15;60(12):1378-1381.

26. Thase ME, Sachs GS. Bipolar depression: pharmacotherapy and related therapeutic strategies. *Biol Psychiatry*. 2000 Sep 15;48(6):558-572.

27. Akiskal HS. "Mood Disorders: Clinical Features." in Sadock BJ, Sadock VA (ed). (2005). *Kaplan & Sadock's Comprehensive Textbook of Psychiatry*. Lippincott Williams & Wilkins:Philadelphia.

28. Sachs GS, Nierenberg AA, Calabrese JR, Marangell LB, Wisniewski SR, Gyulai L, Friedman ES, Bowden CL, Fossey MD, Ostacher MJ, Ketter TA, Patel J, Hauser P, Rapport D, Martinez JM, Allen MH, Miklowitz DJ, Otto MW, Dennehy EB, Thase ME. Effectiveness of adjunctive antidepressant treatment for bipolar depression. *N Engl J Med*. 2007 Apr 26;356(17):1711-1722.

29. MedlinePlus Drug Information: Lithium. http://www.nlm.nih.gov/medlineplus/druginfo/medmaster/a681039.html. Accessed on Nov 19, 2007.

30. MedlinePlus Drug Information: Lamotrigine. http://www.nlm.nih.gov/medlineplus/druginfo/medmaster/a695007.html. Accessed on February 12, 2008.

31. MedlinePlus Drug Information: Valproic Acid. http://www.nlm.nih.gov/medlineplus/druginfo/medmaster/a682412.html. Accessed on February 12, 2008.

32. Lieberman JA, Stroup TS, McEvoy JP, Swartz MS, Rosenheck RA, Perkins DO, Keefe RS, Davis SM, Davis CE, Lebowitz BD, Severe J, Hsiao JK. Effectiveness of antipsychotic drugs in patients with chronic schizophrenia. *N Engl J Med*. 2005 Sep 22;353(12):1209-1223.

33. Nationally Representative CDC Study Finds 1 in 4 Teenage Girls Has a Sexually Transmitted Disease. http://www.cdc.gov/stdconference/2008/media/release-11March2008.htm. Accessed on March 31, 2008.

34. Llewellyn A, Stowe ZN, Strader JR, Jr. The use of lithium and management of women with bipolar disorder during pregnancy and lactation. *J Clin Psychiatry*. 1998 59(Suppl 6):57-64.

35. Yonkers KA, Wisner KL, Stowe Z, Leibenluft E, Cohen L, Miller L, Manber R, Viguera A, Suppes T, Altshuler L. Management of bipolar disorder during pregnancy and the postpartum period. *Am J Psychiatry*. 2004 Apr;161(4):608-620.

36. McClure EB, Treland JE, Snow J, Dickstein DP, Towbin KE, Charney DS, Pine DS, Leibenluft E. Memory and learning in pediatric bipolar disorder. *J Am Acad Child Adolesc Psychiatry*. 2005 May;44(5):461-469.

37. Perlis RH, Ostacher MJ, Patel JK, Marangell LB, Zhang H, Wisniewski SR, Ketter TA, Miklowitz DJ, Otto MW, Gyulai L, Reilly-Harrington NA, Nierenberg AA, Sachs GS, Thase ME. Predictors of recurrence in bipolar disorder: primary outcomes from the Systematic Treatment Enhancement Program for Bipolar Disorder (STEP-BD). *Am J Psychiatry*. 2006 Feb;163(2):217-224.

38. Perlick DA, Rosenheck RA, Clarkin JF, Maciejewski PK, Sirey J, Struening E, Link BG. Impact of family burden and affective response on clinical outcome among patients with bipolar disorder. *Psychiatr Serv*. 2004 Sep;55(9):1029-1035.

For more information on bipolar disorder

Visit the National Library of Medicine's:

MedlinePlus
http://medlineplus.gov

En Español
http://medlineplus.gov/spanish

For information on clinical trials for bipolar disorder:
NIMH supported clinical trials
http://www.nimh.nih.gov/health/trials/index.shtml

National Library of Medicine Clinical Trials Database
http://www.clinicaltrials.gov

Clinical trials at NIMH in Bethesda, MD
http://patientinfo.nimh.nih.gov

Information from NIMH is available in multiple formats. You can browse online, download documents in PDF, and order materials through the mail. Check the NIMH Web site at **http://www.nimh.nih.gov** for the latest information on this topic and to order publications.

If you do not have Internet access please contact the NIMH Information Center at the numbers listed below.

National Institute of Mental Health
Science Writing, Press & Dissemination Branch
6001 Executive Boulevard
Room 8184, MSC 9663
Bethesda, MD 20892-9663
Phone: 301-443-4513 or
1-866-615-NIMH (6464) toll-free
TTY: 301-443-8431
TTY: 866-415-8051 toll-free
FAX: 301-443-4279
E-mail: nimhinfo@nih.gov
Web site: **http://www.nimh.nih.gov**

Reprints:

This publication is in the public domain and may be reproduced or copied without permission from NIMH. We encourage you to reproduce it and use it in your efforts to improve public health. Citation of the National Institute of Mental Health as a source is appreciated. However, using government materials inappropriately can raise legal or ethical concerns, so we ask you to use these guidelines:

- NIMH does not endorse or recommend any commercial products, processes, or services, and our publications may not be used for advertising or endorsement purposes.

- NIMH does not provide specific medical advice or treatment recommendations or referrals; our materials may not be used in a manner that has the appearance of such information.

- NIMH requests that non-Federal organizations not alter our publications in ways that will jeopardize the integrity and "brand" when using the publication.

- Addition of non-Federal Government logos and Web site links may not have the appearance of NIMH endorsement of any specific commercial products or services or medical treatments or services.

If you have questions regarding these guidelines and use of NIMH publications, please contact the NIMH Information Center at 1–866–615–6464 or e-mail at nimhinfo@nih.gov.

The photos in this publication are of models and are used for illustrative purposes only.